HOW TO DEAL
WITH
HEALTH CRISIS

TIPS FOR LONG LIFE

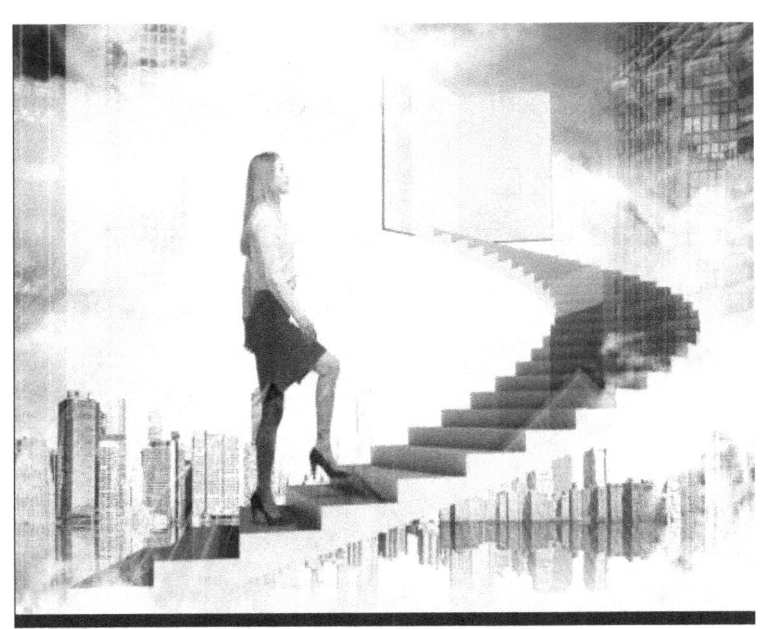

TABLE OF CONTENTS

INTRODUCTION

Once upon a time, there lived a vibrant soul named Emily. She was full of life, always bubbling with energy and enthusiasm. However, one day, a dark cloud loomed over her sunny disposition as she received a diagnosis that shattered her world: cancer. At first, Emily felt like she was drowning in despair. Fear gripped her heart, and uncertainty clouded her thoughts. But deep within her, a tiny spark of resilience flickered. Determined not to let the illness define her, Emily embarked on a journey of healing and self-discovery.

With unwavering determination, Emily faced each chemotherapy session, each painful treatment, with courage and grace. She surrounded herself with love and support from her friends and family, who became her pillars of strength.

As the days turned into weeks and the weeks into months, Emily's spirit refused to be broken. She found solace in the little joys of life – the warmth of the sun on her face, the laughter of her loved ones, and the beauty of each new day.

Slowly but steadily, Emily began to see a glimmer of hope on the horizon. Her body grew stronger, her spirit brighter. She delved into holistic healing practices, embracing yoga, meditation, and healthy eating to nourish her body, mind, and soul.

And then, one miraculous day, the doctors delivered the news she had been praying for – she was cancer-free. Tears of joy streamed down Emily's face as she realized the magnitude of her victory. She had not only survived the darkest chapter of her life but had emerged from it stronger, wiser, and more grateful than ever before.

With a newfound appreciation for the precious gift of life, Emily vowed to live each day to the fullest, spreading love, kindness, and hope wherever she went. Her journey was a testament to the power of resilience, the strength of the human spirit, and the healing force of love. And though she had faced the darkest of storms, Emily emerged as a beacon of light, inspiring all who crossed her path to never give up hope, no matter how daunting the challenge may seem.

CHAPTER 1 : Understanding the Crises

Understanding Health Crises: Causes, Impacts, and Strategies for Addressing Them

Introduction:

Health crises are significant events that disrupt the normal functioning of healthcare systems and pose serious threats to public health. Understanding the complexities surrounding health crises is crucial for effective management and mitigation. This comprehensive content aims to delve into the causes, impacts, and strategies for addressing health crises.

1. Causes of Health Crises:

- Infectious Disease Outbreaks: Epidemics and pandemics caused by pathogens such as viruses, bacteria, and parasites.

- **Natural Disasters**: Events like earthquakes, hurricanes, and floods can lead to injuries, displacement, and increased vulnerability to diseases.

- **Environmental Factors**: Pollution, climate change, and ecological disruptions contribute to health crises by affecting air and water quality, food security, and vector-borne diseases.

- **Socioeconomic Factors**: Poverty, inequality, inadequate healthcare infrastructure, and limited access to essential services exacerbate health crises, particularly in vulnerable populations.

- **Biological Threats**: Emergence of drug-resistant pathogens, bioterrorism, and accidental releases of harmful agents pose serious threats to public health.

2. Impacts of Health Crises:

- **Human Toll**: Loss of life, increased morbidity, psychological trauma, and long-term health consequences for individuals and communities.

- **Economic Burden**: Disruption of businesses, healthcare systems, and supply chains; loss of productivity; healthcare expenditures; and long-term economic consequences.

- **Social Disruption**: Displacement, social unrest, strain on social services, disruption of education, and erosion of trust in institutions.

- **Global Consequences**: Health crises can have far-reaching effects beyond national borders, affecting global trade, travel, and geopolitical dynamics.

3. Strategies for Addressing Health Crises:

- **Prevention and Preparedness**: Investing in surveillance systems, early warning mechanisms, vaccination programs, and disaster preparedness plans.

- **Strengthening Healthcare Systems**: Enhancing healthcare infrastructure, workforce capacity, supply chain resilience, and access to essential services.

- **Risk Communication**: Transparent and timely communication of risks, preventive measures, and healthcare guidelines to the public.

- **Collaboration and Coordination**: Multisectoral collaboration among governments, international organizations, healthcare providers, researchers, and communities.

- **Equity and Inclusion**: Addressing underlying social determinants of health, ensuring access to healthcare for all, and prioritizing the needs of vulnerable populations.

- **Innovation and Research**: Investing in research and development of new diagnostics, treatments, and preventive measures; leveraging technology for healthcare delivery and surveillance.

Conclusion:

Understanding health crises requires a multifaceted approach that encompasses the identification of root causes, assessment of impacts, and implementation of comprehensive strategies for prevention, preparedness, and response. By addressing the underlying determinants of health and fostering global cooperation, we can build more resilient healthcare systems and mitigate the impact of future health crises.

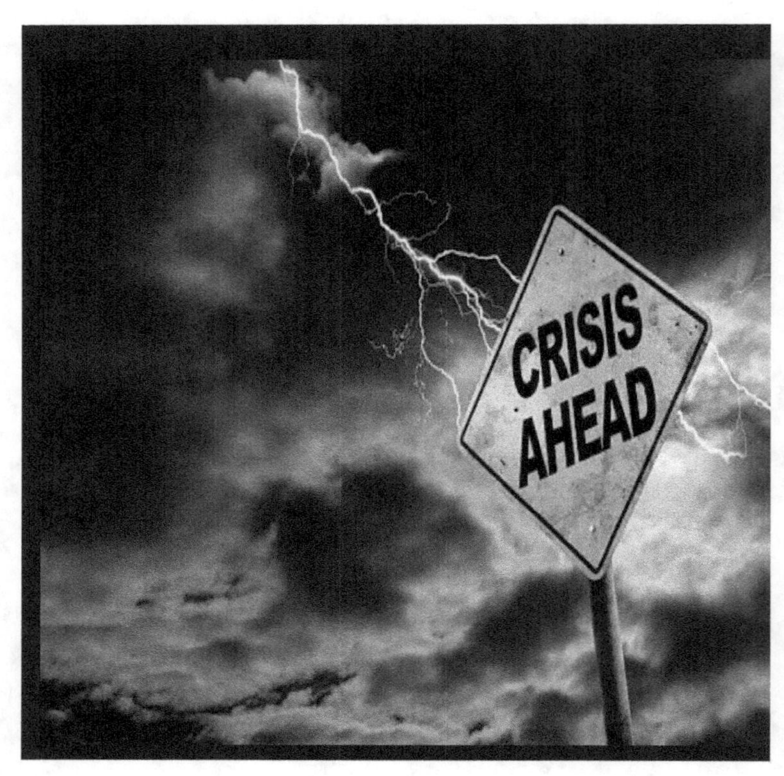
CRISIS
AHEAD

Recognizing Symptoms

Introduction:

Recognizing symptoms is crucial for maintaining good health and addressing potential medical issues before they escalate. Whether it's a sudden onset of pain, changes in appetite, or unusual fatigue, being able to identify and interpret symptoms accurately can lead to timely medical intervention and better health outcomes.

Understanding Symptoms:

Symptoms are the body's way of signaling that something isn't quite right. They can vary widely depending on the underlying cause and individual factors. Symptoms can be categorized into physical, psychological, and behavioral manifestations, each offering valuable clues about a person's health.

Physical Symptoms:

1. Pain: Pain can manifest in various forms, such as dull aches, sharp stabbing sensations, or throbbing discomfort. Its location, intensity, and duration can provide insights into potential underlying conditions.

2. Fatigue: Persistent tiredness or exhaustion that doesn't improve with rest may indicate underlying health issues, including anemia, thyroid disorders, or sleep disorders.

3. Changes in Appearance: Noticeable changes in weight, skin color, or texture can signal nutritional deficiencies, hormonal imbalances, or skin conditions.

4. Digestive Issues: Symptoms like bloating, constipation, diarrhea, or persistent indigestion may point to gastrointestinal disorders or dietary sensitivities.

5. Respiratory Symptoms: Coughing, wheezing, shortness of breath, or chest tightness can be indicative of respiratory infections, allergies, or chronic conditions like asthma.

Psychological Symptoms:

1. Mood Swings: Rapid shifts in mood, persistent sadness, irritability, or feelings of hopelessness may suggest underlying mental health conditions like depression or bipolar disorder.

2. Anxiety: Excessive worry, restlessness, panic attacks, or irrational fears can be signs of anxiety disorders that require professional intervention.

3. Cognitive Changes: Memory loss, confusion, difficulty concentrating, or sudden changes in cognition may indicate neurological conditions such as dementia or Alzheimer's disease.

4. Sleep Disturbances: Insomnia, excessive sleeping, nightmares, or restless sleep patterns can be symptoms of sleep disorders or underlying psychological distress.

Behavioral Symptoms:

1. Changes in Appetite: Significant changes in appetite, including sudden cravings, loss of appetite, or binge eating, can be indicative of underlying physical or mental health issues.

2. Substance Abuse: Increased alcohol consumption, drug use, or addictive behaviors may signal underlying emotional struggles or substance use disorders.

3. Social Withdrawal: Avoidance of social interactions, isolation, or withdrawal from previously enjoyed activities can be red flags for depression, anxiety, or other mental health concerns.

4. Agitation or Aggression: Unexplained irritability, anger outbursts, or hostility may indicate underlying psychological distress or neurological conditions.

Responding to Symptoms:

1. Monitor and Document: Keep track of symptoms, including their frequency, severity, and any associated factors, to provide accurate information to healthcare providers.

2. Seek Medical Advice: Consult a healthcare professional if symptoms persist, worsen, or interfere with daily functioning. Early intervention can prevent complications and improve treatment outcomes.

3. Diagnostic Testing: Healthcare providers may recommend diagnostic tests, such as blood tests, imaging scans, or psychological assessments, to identify the underlying cause of symptoms accurately.

4. Treatment and Management: Follow healthcare provider recommendations for treatment, whether it involves medication, therapy, lifestyle modifications, or a combination of interventions.

5. Self-Care: Adopt healthy lifestyle habits, including regular exercise, balanced nutrition, stress management techniques, and adequate sleep, to support overall well-being and symptom management.

Conclusion:

Recognizing symptoms is the first step towards maintaining good health and addressing potential medical concerns. By understanding the diverse range of symptoms and their potential implications, individuals can take proactive steps to seek appropriate medical care, leading to improved health outcomes and overall quality of life.

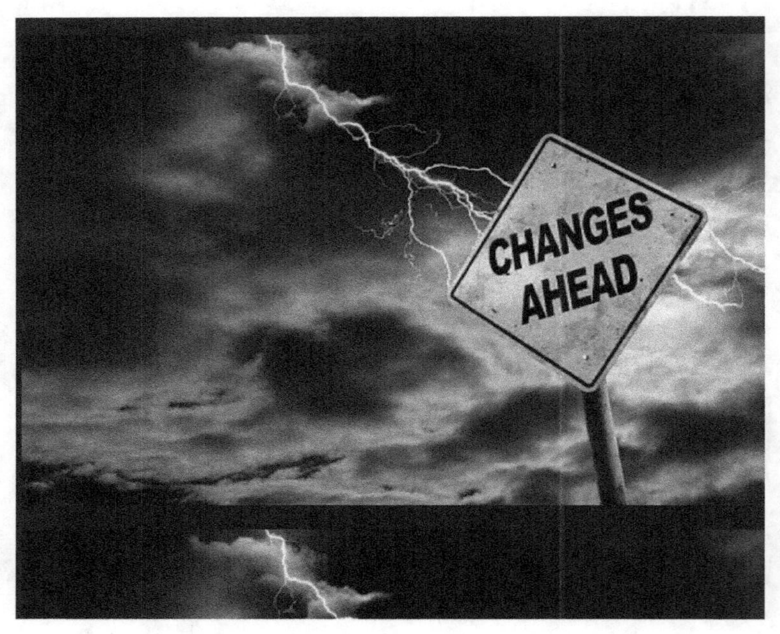
CHANGES
AHEAD

Assessing Severity

Assessing severity is a critical aspect of various fields, including healthcare, emergency response, risk management, and software development. It involves evaluating the magnitude or intensity of an event, situation, or issue to determine its impact and prioritize appropriate actions. Here's a comprehensive guide on assessing severity:

1. Understanding Severity: Severity refers to the extent of harm, damage, or negative consequences resulting from a particular event or condition. It encompasses both the immediate impact and potential long-term implications.

2. Factors Influencing Severity Assessment:

- **Magnitude**: The size, scale, or intensity of the event.

- **Duration**: How long the event lasts or its ongoing effects.

- **Affected Population**: The number of people or entities impacted.

- **Vulnerability**: The susceptibility of affected individuals or systems.

- **Resource Availability**: The availability of resources to mitigate or respond to the event.

- **Context**: The environmental, social, and economic context in which the event occurs.

3. Methods of Assessing Severity:

- **Qualitative Assessment**: Involves subjective judgment based on experience, expertise, and available information. It may include expert opinions, stakeholder consultations, and scenario analysis.

- **Quantitative Assessment**: Involves numerical analysis using metrics, models, or algorithms to measure severity objectively. This may include statistical analysis, mathematical models, and simulations.

- **Risk Assessment**: Evaluates the likelihood and consequences of an event to determine its overall risk severity. It often involves assessing both the probability and impact of potential outcomes.

- **Scenario Planning**: Involves creating hypothetical scenarios to assess the severity of different situations and develop response strategies accordingly.

- **Severity Scales**: Utilizes predefined scales or categories to classify severity levels based on specific criteria. Common examples include the Richter scale for earthquakes and the Saffir-Simpson scale for hurricanes.

4. Tools and Techniques:

- Checklists: Provide a structured approach to assessing severity by systematically evaluating relevant factors.

- **Surveys and Interviews**: Gather input from stakeholders, experts, or affected individuals to understand their perceptions of severity.

- **Data Analysis**: Analyze historical data, trends, and patterns to identify patterns of severity and anticipate future events.

- **Remote Sensing and Monitoring**: Utilize remote sensing technologies and monitoring systems to assess severity in real-time, particularly in environmental and natural disaster contexts.

- **Decision Support Systems**: Use computer-based systems to analyze data and assist decision-making regarding severity assessment and response planning.

5. Applications:

- **Healthcare**: Assessing the severity of illnesses, injuries, or medical conditions to prioritize treatment and allocate resources effectively.

- **Emergency Management**: Evaluating the severity of natural disasters, accidents, or emergencies to coordinate response efforts and allocate resources.

- **Cybersecurity**: Assessing the severity of cybersecurity threats and vulnerabilities to prioritize mitigation efforts and protect critical systems and data.

- **Software Development**: Evaluating the severity of software bugs, errors, or vulnerabilities to prioritize fixes and ensure system reliability and security.

- **Environmental Management**: Assessing the severity of environmental pollution, degradation, or disasters to mitigate impacts and implement remediation measures.

6. Challenges and Considerations:

- **Subjectivity**: Assessing severity often involves subjective judgment, which can introduce biases and inconsistencies.

- **Uncertainty**: There may be uncertainties in the available data, making it challenging to accurately assess severity.

- **Interconnectedness**: Events and their severity may be interconnected, requiring a holistic approach to assessment.

- **Dynamic Nature**: Severity can change over time, requiring continuous monitoring and reassessment.

- **Ethical Considerations**: Assessing severity may involve ethical considerations, such as fairness in resource allocation and decision-making.

7. Response and Mitigation Strategies:

- **Prioritization**: Allocate resources based on the severity of events to address the most critical needs first.

- **Preparedness**: Develop response plans and mitigation strategies tailored to different severity levels.

- Resilience Building: Enhance resilience to reduce the severity of impacts and facilitate recovery from adverse events.

- Public Awareness and Education: Educate the public about the severity of potential risks and the importance of preparedness and mitigation measures.

In conclusion, assessing severity is a multifaceted process that involves understanding, analyzing, and responding to the magnitude and impact of events or conditions across various domains. By employing appropriate methods, tools, and strategies, stakeholders can effectively evaluate severity and mitigate its adverse effects.

Introduction:

Health crises are complex phenomena that can have far-reaching consequences on individuals, communities, and entire nations. Identifying the underlying causes of these crises is essential for developing effective strategies to mitigate their impact and prevent future occurrences. This comprehensive guide aims to explore the various factors that contribute to health crises, from individual behaviors to systemic issues, and provide insights into how to address these root causes.

1. Understanding Health Crises:

- **Definition and Types**: Define what constitutes a health crisis, including epidemics, pandemics, environmental health hazards, and other public health emergencies.

- **Impact**: Discuss the profound effects of health crises on physical and mental health, socio-economic stability, and healthcare systems.

2. Analyzing the Causes:

a. Biological Factors:

- Infectious Diseases: Explore the role of pathogens such as viruses, bacteria, and parasites in causing epidemics and pandemics.

- **Chronic Conditions**: Discuss how non-communicable diseases contribute to health crises, including obesity, diabetes, and cardiovascular diseases.

b. Behavioral Factors:

- **Lifestyle Choices**: Examine how individual behaviors such as smoking, poor diet, and lack of exercise contribute to the development and spread of health crises.

- **Risky Behaviors**: Address the impact of risky behaviors such as substance abuse and unsafe sexual practices on public health.

c. Environmental Factors:

- **Pollution**: Discuss the effects of air, water, and soil pollution on human health, including respiratory diseases and cancer.

- **Climate Change**: Explore the links between climate change and health crises, including extreme weather events, food insecurity, and the spread of vector-borne diseases.

d. Socio-Economic Factors:

- **Poverty**: Analyze the relationship between poverty and health disparities, including limited access to healthcare, nutritious food, and safe housing.

- **Inequality**: Discuss how social inequalities based on factors such as race, ethnicity, gender, and socioeconomic status contribute to health inequities.

e. Healthcare System Factors:

- **Access and Quality**: Address the challenges related to healthcare access, affordability, and quality, particularly in underserved communities.

- Infrastructure: Examine the role of healthcare infrastructure, including hospitals, clinics, and public health agencies, in responding to health crises.

3. Addressing Root Causes:

- **Prevention Strategies**: Propose preventive measures targeting the root causes of health crises, including public health education, behavior change interventions, and environmental regulations.

- **Health Equity**: Advocate for policies and programs aimed at reducing health disparities and promoting health equity, such as expanding access to healthcare services and addressing social determinants of health.

- **Preparedness and Response**: Highlight the importance of building robust healthcare systems and emergency preparedness plans to effectively respond to health crises when they occur.

- **Research and Innovation**: Emphasize the need for continued research and innovation in public health, medicine, and technology to better understand and address the root causes of health crises.

Conclusion:

Identifying the causes of health crises requires a multifaceted approach that considers biological, behavioral, environmental, socio-economic, and healthcare system factors. By understanding the root causes and implementing comprehensive strategies to address them, we can work towards building healthier, more resilient communities and preventing future health crises.

CHAPTER 2: Seeking Immediate Assistance

Introduction:

In times of health crises, knowing how to seek immediate assistance can make all the difference between life and death. Whether it's a sudden injury, a severe illness, or a mental health emergency, having a clear plan of action and knowing where to turn for help is crucial. This comprehensive guide aims to provide you with the necessary information and resources to navigate through such challenging situations effectively.

1. Recognizing the Signs of a Health Crisis:

- **Physical Health Crisis**: Symptoms such as severe pain, difficulty breathing, chest pain, excessive bleeding, loss of consciousness, or sudden weakness should never be ignored.

- **Mental Health Crisis**: Signs may include extreme mood swings, thoughts of self-harm or suicide, hallucinations, paranoia, or sudden changes in behavior.

2. Immediate Actions to Take:

- **Call Emergency Services**: In case of a medical emergency, dial the emergency services number (e.g., 911 in the United States) immediately.

- **Provide Necessary Information**: Clearly communicate the nature of the emergency, the location, and any relevant medical history.

- **Stay Calm and Provide Basic First Aid**: If safe to do so, administer basic first aid while waiting for emergency responders.

3. Utilizing Emergency Medical Services (EMS):

- **Ambulance Services**: EMS can dispatch ambulances equipped with medical professionals and necessary equipment to provide immediate medical care en route to the hospital.

- **Paramedics and Emergency Medical Technicians (EMTs)**: These trained professionals can administer life-saving interventions on-site and during transportation to the hospital.

4. Contacting Healthcare Providers:

- **Primary Care Physician**: If the situation is urgent but not immediately life-threatening, contact your primary care physician or their after-hours service for guidance.

- **Specialist Care**: For specific health crises related to ongoing conditions, contact relevant specialists or disease-specific hotlines for assistance.

5. Seeking Mental Health Support:

- **Crisis Hotlines**: Mental health crisis hotlines provide immediate support and guidance for individuals experiencing emotional distress or suicidal thoughts.

- **Mobile Crisis Teams**: Many communities have mobile crisis teams consisting of mental health professionals who can provide on-site assessment and intervention.

6. Utilizing Telehealth Services:

- **Telemedicine Platforms**: In non-life-threatening situations, telemedicine services allow individuals to consult with healthcare professionals remotely via video calls or phone consultations.

- **Mental Health Apps**: There are various apps and online platforms offering therapy, counseling, and mental health resources accessible from the comfort of home.

7. Additional Resources and Support:

- **Community Health Centers**: Local health centers often offer a range of medical and mental health services, including sliding-scale fees for those without insurance.

- **Support Groups**: Connecting with support groups or online communities can provide valuable peer support and resources for coping with health crises.

Conclusion:

Navigating a health crisis can be overwhelming, but knowing how to seek immediate assistance is crucial for ensuring timely and appropriate care. By recognizing the signs of a health crisis, taking immediate actions, and utilizing available resources and support networks, individuals can effectively manage emergencies and access the care they need when it matters most.

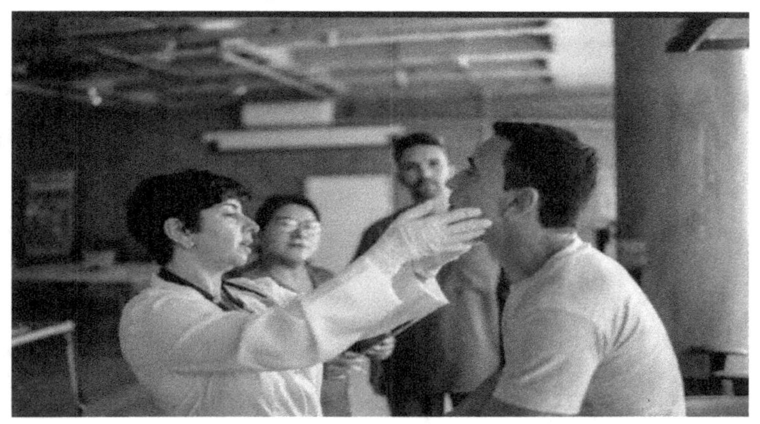

Emergency Hotlines

Introduction:

In times of health crisis, having access to emergency hotlines can be crucial for receiving immediate assistance and guidance. Whether it's a medical emergency, mental health crisis, or any other health-related concern, knowing the appropriate hotline to call can save lives. This comprehensive guide provides an overview of various emergency hotlines for different health crises, ensuring that individuals can quickly access the help they need when it matters most.

1. Medical Emergencies:

- **911 (United States and Canada)**: This is the universal emergency number for immediate assistance in case of medical emergencies, accidents, fires, or any life-threatening situation. Calling 911 connects you to emergency medical services (EMS), who dispatch paramedics or other emergency responders to your location.

- **112 (European Union and various other countries)**: Similar to 911, 112 is the emergency number for medical, fire, and police emergencies in many countries across Europe and other regions.

- **999 (United Kingdom)**: In the UK, 999 is the emergency number for contacting ambulance, fire, police, and coastguard services for immediate assistance.

2. Mental Health Crisis:

- National Suicide Prevention Lifeline (US): 1-800-273-TALK (8255) - Provides free and confidential support for individuals in distress, including those having suicidal thoughts. Trained counselors are available 24/7 to provide support and connect callers to local resources.

- Crisis Text Line (US): Text HOME to 741741 - Offers free, confidential support via text message for anyone in crisis, including thoughts of suicide, anxiety, depression, or any other mental health concern.

- Samaritans (UK): 116 123 - Provides confidential emotional support for individuals experiencing feelings of distress or despair, including those having suicidal thoughts. Available 24/7, callers can talk to trained volunteers who offer non-judgmental listening and support.

3. Substance Abuse and Addiction:

- **SAMHSA National Helpline (US)**: 1-800-662-HELP (4357) - Offers free, confidential treatment referral and information for individuals and families facing substance abuse and mental health disorders. Available 24/7, in English and Spanish.

- **National Drug Helpline (UK):** 0300 123 6600 - Provides confidential support, advice, and information for individuals struggling with drug addiction and substance abuse. Trained advisors offer guidance on treatment options and local support services.

4. Domestic Violence and Abuse:

- National Domestic Violence Hotline (US): 1-800-799-SAFE (7233) - Offers support, crisis intervention, safety planning, and resources for individuals experiencing domestic violence or abuse. Available 24/7, confidential, and multilingual.

- National Domestic Abuse Helpline (UK): 0808 2000 247 - Provides confidential support, information, and guidance for individuals experiencing domestic abuse. Available 24/7, callers can speak to trained advisors who offer emotional support and practical assistance.

Conclusion:

Having access to emergency hotlines for various health crises is essential for ensuring prompt assistance and support when needed. Whether it's a medical emergency, mental health crisis, substance abuse issue, or domestic violence situation, these hotlines offer confidential support, guidance, and resources to individuals in distress. It's important to familiarize yourself with these hotlines and share this information with others to promote health and safety in our communities.

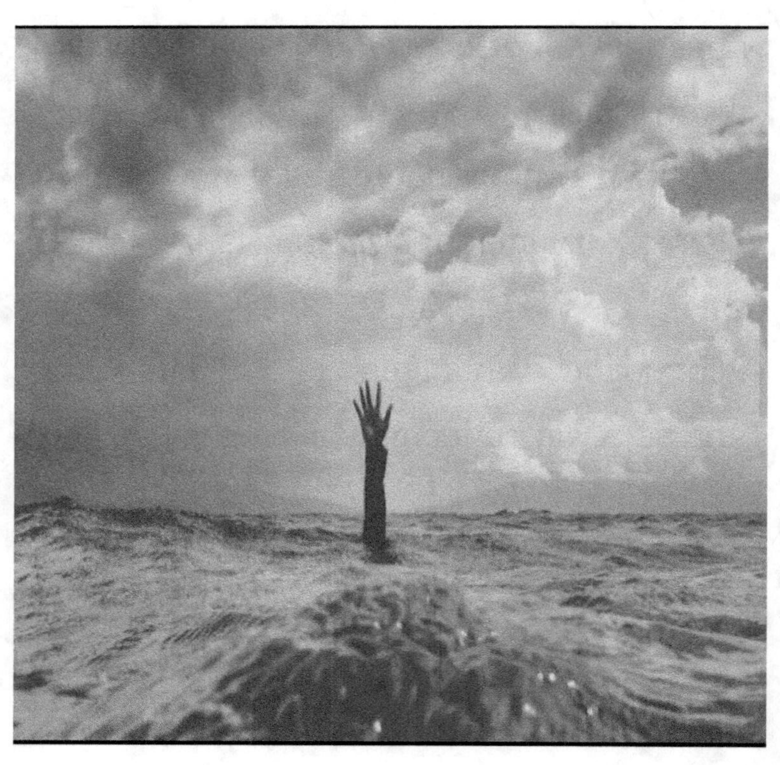

Nearby Medical Facilities

Introduction:

In times of medical emergencies or routine healthcare needs, having access to nearby medical facilities is crucial. Whether you're new to an area or simply seeking to familiarize yourself with the available healthcare options, this guide will provide comprehensive insights into navigating nearby medical facilities.

1. Understanding Medical Facility Types:

- **Hospitals**: Typically equipped to handle a wide range of medical emergencies and provide specialized care.

- **Urgent Care Centers**: Offer immediate medical attention for non-life-threatening conditions when primary care physicians are unavailable.

- **Clinics**: Provide outpatient services, including routine check-ups, vaccinations, and minor procedures.

- **Pharmacies**: Offer prescription medications, over-the-counter drugs, and sometimes basic health services like vaccinations and health screenings.

2. Researching Nearby Medical Facilities:

- **Utilize online resources**: Websites and apps like Google Maps, Yelp, or dedicated healthcare directories provide information on nearby medical facilities, including ratings, reviews, and services offered.

- **Consult healthcare providers**: Primary care physicians or local health departments can offer recommendations based on your specific healthcare needs.

3. Evaluating Services Offered:

- **Emergency Services**: Determine if the facility offers emergency medical care, including trauma care, intensive care, and emergency surgeries.

- **Specialized Care**: Look for facilities that provide specialized services such as cardiology, orthopedics, obstetrics, and pediatrics.

- **Diagnostic Services**: Check if the facility offers imaging services (X-rays, MRI, CT scans) and laboratory testing for accurate diagnoses.

- **Ancillary Services**: Consider additional services like physical therapy, pharmacy, and mental health counseling available on-site.

4. Assessing Quality and Reputation:

- **Accreditation**: Verify if the facility is accredited by recognized organizations such as The Joint Commission or the Accreditation Commission for Healthcare.

- **Patient Reviews**: Read patient reviews and testimonials to gauge the overall quality of care, cleanliness, staff friendliness, and wait times.

- **Clinical Outcomes**: Look for data on clinical outcomes and patient safety measures to assess the facility's performance.

5. Accessibility and Convenience:

- **Location**: Choose facilities that are easily accessible from your home, workplace, or frequently visited areas.

- **Operating Hours**: Consider the facility's hours of operation, including evenings, weekends, and holidays, to accommodate your schedule.

- **Transportation**: Assess transportation options available to reach the facility, including public transportation, parking availability, and proximity to major roadways.

6. Emergency Preparedness:

- **Disaster Response**: Inquire about the facility's protocols for handling natural disasters, pandemics, or mass casualty incidents.

- **Medical Equipment**: Ensure the facility is equipped with essential medical supplies, emergency generators, and backup systems to maintain operations during emergencies.

Conclusion:

Navigating nearby medical facilities requires thorough research, evaluation of services, consideration of quality and reputation, assessment of accessibility, and awareness of emergency preparedness. By leveraging the information and resources provided in this guide, individuals can make informed decisions to access timely and quality healthcare when needed.

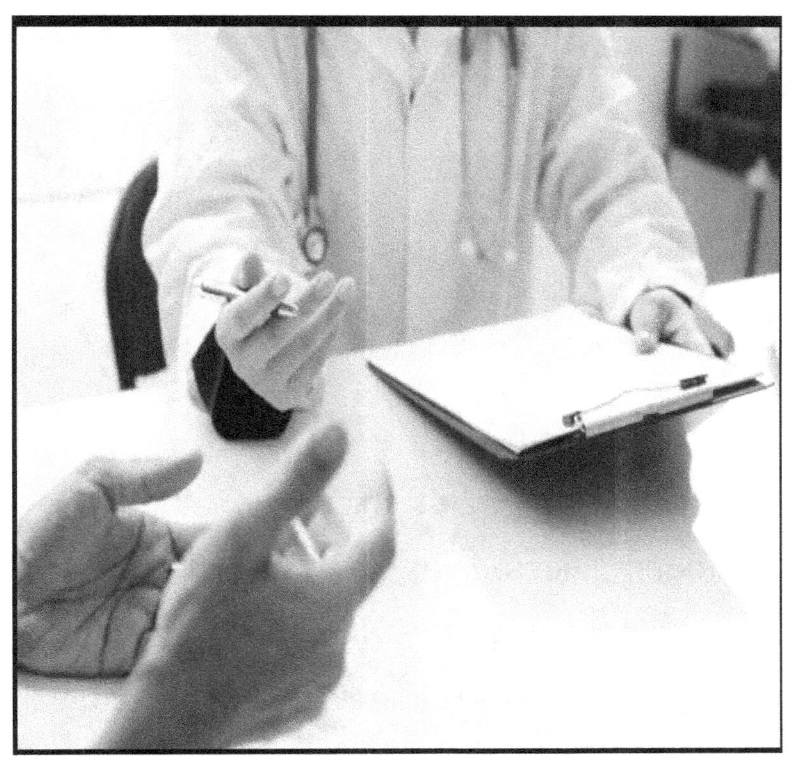

Contacting Healthcare Professionals

Introduction:

In times of health crises, whether it's a sudden illness, injury, or worsening chronic condition, knowing how to effectively contact healthcare professionals can be crucial. This comprehensive guide aims to provide you with the necessary information and steps to reach out to healthcare professionals promptly and efficiently during a health emergency.

1. Assess the Situation:

- Before contacting healthcare professionals, assess the severity of the situation. Is it an emergency requiring immediate medical attention, or can it be addressed through other means?

- If the situation is life-threatening, call emergency services immediately (e.g., 911 in the United States, 999 in the United Kingdom, 112 in Europe).

2. Primary Care Physician:

- If the situation is urgent but not life-threatening, contact your primary care physician first.

- Most primary care physicians have after-hours protocols for emergencies. Follow their instructions on how to reach them or their on-call service.

3. Specialist Physicians:

- For ongoing conditions or specialized care, contact your specialist physician directly.

- Keep a list of your specialist physicians and their contact information handy for easy reference during emergencies.

4. Urgent Care Centers:

- If your primary care physician is unavailable, consider visiting an urgent care center for non-life-threatening emergencies.

- Urgent care centers can provide prompt medical attention for a wide range of conditions, including minor injuries and illnesses.

5. Telehealth Services:

- In non-emergency situations or for medical advice, consider utilizing telehealth services.

- Many healthcare providers offer virtual consultations, allowing you to speak with a healthcare professional from the comfort of your home.

6. Hospital Emergency Departments:

- If the situation is critical or life-threatening, proceed directly to the nearest hospital emergency department.

- Emergency departments are equipped to handle a wide range of medical emergencies and operate 24/7.

7. Medical Hotlines:

- Some regions have medical hotlines staffed by healthcare professionals who can provide advice and guidance over the phone.

- These hotlines can be valuable resources for obtaining medical information and determining the appropriate course of action.

8. Family and Friends:

- In situations where you are unable to contact healthcare professionals yourself, enlist the help of family members or friends.

- They can assist in making phone calls, arranging transportation, and providing support during medical emergencies.

9. Keep Important Information Handy:

- Maintain a list of important medical information, including medications, allergies, and past medical history.

- Store this information in a readily accessible location, such as a wallet or smartphone, to provide to healthcare professionals when needed.

10. Follow-Up Care:

- After receiving initial treatment or advice, follow up with your healthcare provider as necessary.

- Attend scheduled appointments, adhere to prescribed medications, and communicate any changes in your condition promptly.

Conclusion:

In times of health crisis, knowing how to contact healthcare professionals efficiently can make a significant difference in the outcome. By following the steps outlined in this comprehensive guide and staying prepared, you can ensure timely access to medical care and support when it's needed most. Remember, prioritizing your health and safety is paramount, so don't hesitate to seek help when faced with a medical emergency.

CHAPTER 3: Staying Calm and Collected

Introduction:

In times of health crises, such as pandemics or personal health emergencies, maintaining a sense of calm and composure is paramount. Despite the uncertainty and anxiety that often accompany such situations, staying level-headed can greatly improve decision-making, overall well-being, and resilience. Here, we explore various strategies and techniques to help individuals remain composed during health crises.

Understanding the Situation:

1. Educate Yourself: Stay informed about the health crisis through credible sources to understand the facts, risks, and necessary precautions. Knowledge can alleviate fear and empower you to make informed decisions.

2. Perspective Shift: Remind yourself that while the situation may be challenging, it is temporary and manageable. Focus on what you can control, such as following health guidelines and taking care of yourself and your loved ones.

3. Acceptance: Acknowledge your emotions without judgment. It's normal to feel anxious, scared, or overwhelmed during a health crisis. Accepting these feelings can help you process them and move forward with a clearer mindset.

Practicing Self-Care:

1. Mindfulness and Meditation: Engage in mindfulness practices or meditation to cultivate inner peace and reduce stress. Even a few minutes of deep breathing or guided meditation can help center your mind amidst chaos.

2. **Healthy Habits**: Prioritize self-care activities like regular exercise, nutritious eating, and sufficient sleep. Physical well-being directly impacts mental resilience, making it easier to stay calm in challenging situations.

3. **Limit Media Exposure**: While staying informed is important, excessive exposure to distressing news can fuel anxiety and panic. Set boundaries on media consumption and take breaks to focus on uplifting or distracting activities.

Building a Support System:

1. Connect with Others: Lean on your support network, whether it's friends, family, or online communities. Sharing your concerns and experiences can provide comfort and reassurance, reminding you that you're not alone in facing the crisis.

2. Seek Professional Help: If you're struggling to cope with anxiety or stress, consider reaching out to a therapist or counselor. Professional support can offer valuable coping strategies and emotional guidance tailored to your needs.

3. Offer Support to Others: Helping others in need can foster a sense of purpose and connection, counteracting feelings of helplessness. Whether it's checking in on a neighbor or volunteering for relief efforts, contributing positively can boost your own resilience.

Practical Coping Strategies:

1. Develop a Routine: Establishing a daily routine can provide structure and stability during uncertain times. Set specific goals and tasks to focus on, breaking down overwhelming situations into manageable steps.

2. Practice Relaxation Techniques: Experiment with relaxation techniques such as progressive muscle relaxation, visualization, or aromatherapy. Find what works best for you and incorporate it into your daily routine to promote calmness and relaxation.

3. Stay Flexible: Flexibility is key in navigating unpredictable situations. Be prepared to adapt your plans and expectations as circumstances change, focusing on solutions rather than dwelling on setbacks.

Conclusion:

In the face of health crises, maintaining composure is a valuable skill that can foster resilience and well-being. By understanding the situation, practicing self-care, building a support system, and implementing practical coping strategies, individuals can navigate challenging times with grace and resilience. Remember, staying calm and collected isn't about suppressing emotions, but rather about managing them effectively to make sound decisions and maintain mental well-being.

Managing Panic

In times of health crises, such as epidemics or outbreaks, managing panic is crucial for maintaining individual and collective well-being. Panic can exacerbate the situation, lead to irrational decision-making, and spread misinformation. Here's a comprehensive guide on how to manage panic effectively during health crises:

1. Stay Informed, but Limit Exposure: Stay updated with information from reliable sources such as the World Health Organization (WHO), Centers for Disease Control and Prevention (CDC), or local health authorities. However, limit exposure to news and social media to avoid feeling overwhelmed by sensationalized or inaccurate information.

2. Focus on Facts, Not Fear: Stick to facts and evidence-based information. Avoid rumors and unverified information circulating on social media. Verify information before sharing it with others to prevent the spread of misinformation.

3. Maintain a Routine: Stick to a regular routine as much as possible. Establishing a sense of normalcy can help reduce anxiety and provide a sense of control amid uncertainty.

4. Practice Self-Care: Take care of your physical and mental health. Get enough sleep, eat nutritious meals, exercise regularly, and practice relaxation techniques such as deep breathing or meditation to reduce stress.

5. Stay Connected: Stay connected with friends and family members through phone calls, video chats, or social media. Share your concerns and feelings with trusted individuals, and offer support to others who may be struggling.

6. Limit Exposure to Negative Influences: Avoid conversations or interactions that fuel panic or anxiety. Surround yourself with positive influences and supportive individuals who can help you stay grounded and calm.

7. Engage in Meaningful Activities: Engage in activities that bring you joy and fulfillment, whether it's reading, listening to music, cooking, or pursuing a hobby.

Distracting yourself with enjoyable activities can help alleviate stress and anxiety.

8. Seek Reliable Support: If you're feeling overwhelmed by anxiety or panic, don't hesitate to seek support from a mental health professional. Many therapists offer remote sessions via phone or video chat, making it easier to access support during a health crisis.

9. Follow Recommended Precautions: Take practical steps to protect yourself and others from infection, such as washing your hands frequently, wearing a mask in public settings, and practicing physical distancing. Following these precautions can help alleviate anxiety by empowering you to take proactive measures.

10. Focus on What You Can Control: Focus on the aspects of the situation that you can control, such as following recommended guidelines, practicing good hygiene, and supporting others in your community. Let go of worry about things beyond your control.

11. Stay Flexible and Adaptive: Understand that the situation may evolve rapidly, and plans may need to change accordingly. Stay flexible and adaptive in your approach, and be prepared to adjust your routines and behaviors as needed.

12. Limit Substance Use: Avoid using alcohol, drugs, or other substances as a coping mechanism for anxiety or stress. While they may provide temporary relief, they can exacerbate mental health issues and impair judgment.

By implementing these strategies, you can effectively manage panic and anxiety during health crises, while also contributing to a sense of collective resilience and solidarity within your community. Remember, it's normal to feel anxious or overwhelmed during challenging times, but by taking proactive steps to care for yourself and others, you can navigate the situation with greater calm and confidence.

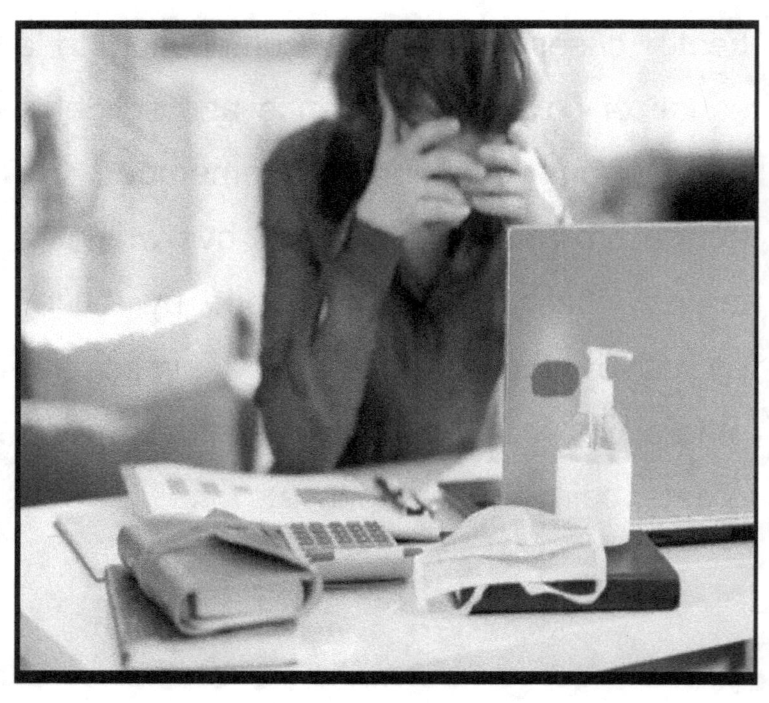

Supporting Loved Ones

Introduction:

Health crises can be emotionally and physically challenging for both the individual experiencing them and their loved ones. Providing support during these times is crucial for maintaining the well-being of everyone involved. This comprehensive guide aims to offer practical advice and strategies for supporting loved ones through health crises.

1. Understanding the Situation:

- **Communicate openly**: Encourage open and honest communication to understand the nature and severity of the health crisis.

- **Educate yourself**: Learn about the condition or illness to better understand its implications and how you can offer support.

- **Respect privacy**: Respect your loved one's privacy and boundaries while offering your support.

2. Emotional Support:

- **Be empathetic**: Show empathy and understanding towards your loved one's feelings and emotions.

- **Listen actively**: Allow your loved one to express their fears, concerns, and emotions without judgment.

- **Offer reassurance**: Provide words of comfort and reassurance to alleviate anxiety and stress.

- **Seek professional help**: Encourage your loved one to seek professional support from therapists or counselors if needed.

3. Practical Support:

- **Assist with daily tasks**: Offer assistance with daily chores, errands, and responsibilities to alleviate stress.

- **Coordinate medical appointments**: Help organize and accompany your loved one to medical appointments, and take notes during consultations.

- **Provide transportation**: Offer transportation to and from medical facilities or appointments if needed.

- **Help with medication management**: Assist in organizing and managing medications to ensure adherence to treatment plans.

4. Maintain Normalcy:

- **Encourage normal activities**: Encourage your loved one to engage in activities they enjoy to maintain a sense of normalcy.

- **Spend quality time together**: Plan activities or spend quality time together to strengthen your bond and provide a sense of comfort.

- **Foster a positive environment**: Create a positive and uplifting atmosphere by surrounding your loved one with supportive friends and family members.

- **Practice self-care**: Take care of your own physical and emotional well-being to better support your loved one effectively.

5. Financial Support:

- Offer financial assistance: Provide financial support if needed, such as helping with medical bills or expenses related to treatment.

- **Explore resources**: Research financial assistance programs, grants, or community resources that may offer support during this time.

- **Assist with insurance**: Help navigate insurance policies and claims to ensure coverage for medical expenses.

6. Stay Informed and Adaptive:

- **Stay updated**: Stay informed about your loved one's condition, treatment options, and progress.

- **Be flexible**: Be prepared to adapt to changes in the situation and provide support accordingly.

- **Advocate for your loved one**: Advocate for your loved one's needs and preferences within the healthcare system to ensure they receive the best possible care.

Conclusion:

Supporting a loved one through a health crisis requires patience, empathy, and resilience. By understanding their needs, offering emotional and practical support, maintaining normalcy, providing financial assistance when necessary, and staying informed and adaptive, you can help your loved one navigate through this challenging time with strength and dignity. Remember, your presence and support can make a significant difference in their journey towards recovery.

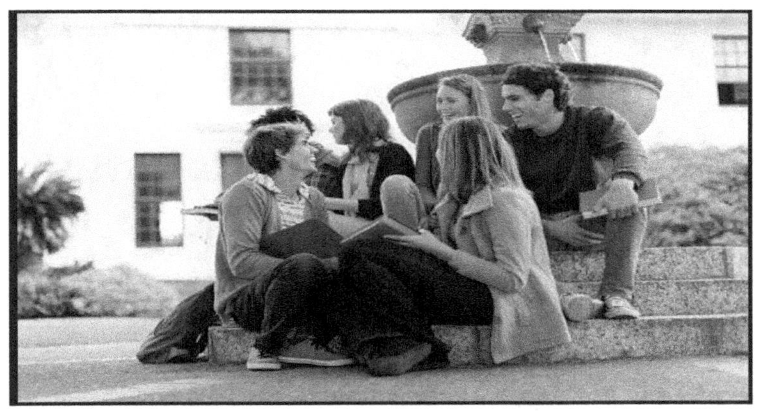

CHAPTER 4 : Taking Immediate Action

Introduction:

In times of health crises, swift and effective action is paramount to mitigate the impact and save lives. Whether it's a pandemic, natural disaster, or localized outbreak, taking immediate action requires a well-coordinated approach involving various stakeholders. This comprehensive guide outlines strategies and steps to tackle health crises promptly and efficiently.

1. Assessment and Risk Analysis:

- Evaluate the nature and scope of the health crisis.

- Conduct a risk analysis to understand potential threats and vulnerabilities.

- Gather data on affected populations, transmission patterns, and resource availability.

2. Communication and Coordination:

- Establish clear communication channels among relevant authorities, healthcare providers, and the public.

- Ensure accurate and timely dissemination of information to prevent misinformation and panic.

- Coordinate efforts between local, national, and international organizations for a unified response.

3. Mobilizing Resources:

- Allocate sufficient financial, human, and material resources to address immediate needs.

- Secure medical supplies, equipment, and facilities for diagnosis, treatment, and containment.

- Activate emergency response teams and establish temporary healthcare facilities if necessary.

4. Implementing Public Health Measures:

- Enforce preventive measures such as vaccination campaigns, hygiene promotion, and social distancing.

- Implement surveillance systems for early detection and monitoring of cases.

- Enact travel restrictions and quarantine measures to limit the spread of infectious diseases.

5. Healthcare Capacity Enhancement:

- Expand healthcare capacity by increasing the number of beds, medical staff, and testing facilities.

- Train healthcare workers on infection control protocols and treatment guidelines.

- Develop protocols for triage, patient management, and referral systems to optimize care delivery.

6. Community Engagement and Support:

- Engage with communities to build trust, address concerns, and promote cooperation.

- Provide support services for vulnerable populations, including access to healthcare, food, and shelter.

- Foster partnerships with local organizations and community leaders to facilitate outreach and response efforts.

7. Monitoring and Evaluation:

- Continuously monitor the progress of interventions and adapt strategies based on emerging trends.

- Conduct regular evaluations to assess the effectiveness of response activities and identify areas for improvement.

- Share lessons learned and best practices to strengthen preparedness for future health crises.

8. Sustainability and Long-term Planning:

- Develop sustainable strategies for maintaining preparedness and resilience in the face of future health threats.

- Invest in research and development of new technologies, treatments, and vaccines.

- Advocate for policies that prioritize public health, equity, and disaster risk reduction.

Conclusion:

Taking immediate action on health crises requires a multifaceted approach that encompasses assessment, communication, resource mobilization, public health measures, capacity enhancement, community engagement, monitoring, and long-term planning. By implementing these strategies and steps effectively, governments, organizations, and communities can mitigate the impact of health crises and protect the well-being of populations worldwide.

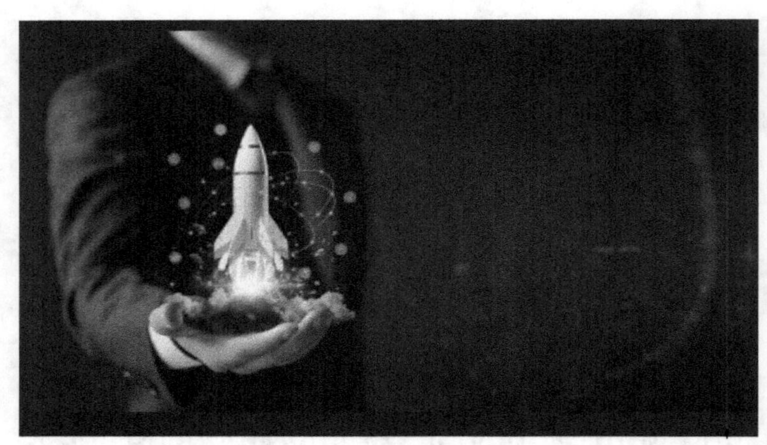

First Aid Measures

Introduction:

In times of health crises, knowing how to administer first aid can be crucial in providing immediate assistance to those in need. Whether it's a natural disaster, a sudden medical emergency, or a public health outbreak, being prepared with the right first aid measures can save lives. This comprehensive guide aims to equip individuals with the knowledge and skills necessary to respond effectively during health crisis situations.

Section 1: Preparedness

1.1. Emergency Preparedness Kit:

- List essential items such as bandages, antiseptic wipes, gloves, medications, and emergency contact information.

1.2. Emergency Plan:

- Develop a plan outlining evacuation routes, meeting points, and communication methods.

1.3. Training and Certification:

- Encourage individuals to undergo first aid and CPR training courses to acquire necessary skills and knowledge.

Section 2: Basic First Aid Techniques

2.1. Assessing the Situation:

- Prioritize safety for both the responder and the victim.

2.2. ABCs of First Aid:

- **Airway**: Ensure the airway is clear.

- **Breathing**: Check for breathing.

- **Circulation**: Assess pulse and control bleeding if present.

2.3. CPR (Cardiopulmonary Resuscitation):

- Provide step-by-step instructions for performing CPR on adults, children, and infants.

2.4. Choking:

- Outline the Heimlich maneuver for conscious and unconscious individuals.

2.5. Bleeding Control:

- Demonstrate how to apply direct pressure, elevate the wound, and use pressure points if necessary.

2.6. Shock Management:

- Explain the signs and symptoms of shock and appropriate first aid measures.

Section 3: Specific Health Crisis Scenarios

3.1. Natural Disasters:

- Address common injuries such as cuts, fractures, and hypothermia.

3.2. Infectious Disease Outbreaks:

- Provide guidance on personal protective measures, isolation protocols, and symptoms recognition.

3.3. Medical Emergencies:

- Include first aid measures for heart attacks, strokes, seizures, and allergic reactions.

Section 4: Psychological First Aid

4.1. Emotional Support:

- Offer tips for providing comfort and reassurance to individuals experiencing distress.

4.2. Active Listening:

- Emphasize the importance of listening empathetically and without judgment.

4.3. Referral to Professional Help:

- Provide information on local mental health resources and support services.

Conclusion:

Being equipped with the knowledge and skills to administer first aid during health crisis situations is invaluable. By following the guidelines outlined in this comprehensive content, individuals can play a vital role in mitigating the impact of emergencies and providing immediate assistance to those in need. Remember, preparedness and quick action can make all the difference in saving lives.

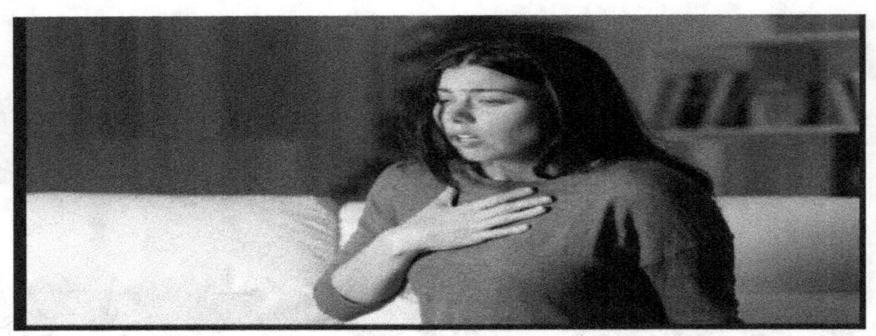

Introduction:

Administering medications is a critical aspect of healthcare delivery, requiring precision, caution, and expertise. Whether it's oral medications, injections, or intravenous infusions, proper administration is vital for patient safety and effective treatment outcomes. This comprehensive guide aims to provide healthcare professionals with essential knowledge and best practices for administering medications.

1. Understanding Medications:

- Different types of medications: oral, topical, parenteral (injections), inhalation, etc.

- Pharmacokinetics and pharmacodynamics: absorption, distribution, metabolism, and excretion.

- **Drug classifications**: analgesics, antibiotics, anticoagulants, etc.

- Importance of medication reconciliation and verifying prescriptions.

2. Preparing for Medication Administration:

- Reviewing a patient's medical history, allergies, and current medications.

- Ensuring correct dosage and medication form.

- Gathering necessary equipment: syringes, needles, IV tubing, etc.

- Following aseptic techniques to prevent contamination.

3. Oral Medication Administration:

- Techniques for administering tablets, capsules, liquids, and sublingual medications.

- Ensuring patient understanding of dosage and administration instructions.

- Documenting medication administration accurately.

4. Parenteral Medication Administration:

- Subcutaneous, intramuscular, and intravenous injection techniques.

- Needle selection based on patient's age, weight, and medication viscosity.

- Safe disposal of needles and sharps.

5. Intravenous Medication Administration:

- Proper IV site selection and catheter insertion.

- Calculating drip rates and monitoring infusion rates.

- Preventing complications such as infiltration, phlebitis, and air embolism.

6. Topical and Transdermal Medication **Administration**:

- Application techniques for creams, ointments, patches, and gels.

- Skin preparation and site rotation for transdermal patches.

- Monitoring for skin reactions and absorption rates.

7. Inhalation Medication Administration:

- Proper use of metered-dose inhalers (MDIs) and dry powder inhalers (DPIs).

- Teaching patients correct inhalation techniques.

- Cleaning and maintenance of inhalation devices.

8. Special Considerations:

- Pediatric and geriatric medication administration.

- Patients with swallowing difficulties or impaired cognitive function.

- Cultural and language considerations in medication education.

9. Monitoring and Evaluation:

- Assessing patient response to medications.

- Monitoring for adverse reactions and drug interactions.

- Documenting medication administration and patient outcomes.

10. Patient Education:

- Providing clear instructions on medication use, side effects, and precautions.

- Encouraging adherence to medication regimen.

- Addressing patient concerns and questions.

Conclusion:

Administering medications is a multifaceted responsibility that requires attention to detail, clinical competence, and compassionate care. By following best practices, healthcare professionals can ensure safe and effective medication administration, promoting positive patient outcomes and quality of care.

CHAPTER 5: Communication and Documentation

Introduction:

Communication and documentation are foundational elements in virtually every aspect of human interaction, from personal relationships to professional endeavors. In fields such as business, healthcare, education, and technology, effective communication and meticulous documentation play critical roles in ensuring clarity, efficiency, accountability, and compliance. This guide explores the importance of communication and documentation, their key principles, best practices, and their significance across various domains.

1. Importance of Communication:

- Facilitates Understanding: Effective communication fosters clear understanding among individuals or groups, minimizing misunderstandings and conflicts.

- **Builds Relationships**: Strong communication skills are essential for building and maintaining healthy relationships, both personally and professionally.

- **Enhances Collaboration**: Clear and open communication encourages collaboration, creativity, and innovation within teams and organizations.

- **Drives Success**: Effective communication is often cited as a key driver of success in business, leadership, and personal development.

- **Improves Problem-Solving**: Clear communication enables individuals to articulate problems, exchange ideas, and collaborate on solutions more efficiently.

2. Principles of Effective Communication:

- **Clarity**: Messages should be clear, concise, and easily understood by the intended audience.

- **Active Listening**: Listening attentively to others fosters mutual understanding and empathy.

- **Empathy**: Understanding others' perspectives and feelings promotes effective communication and relationship-building.

- **Feedback**: Providing and receiving constructive feedback is essential for continuous improvement and growth.

- **Adaptability**: Adapting communication style to suit different situations and audiences enhances effectiveness.

3. Modes of Communication:

- **Verbal Communication**: Involves speaking and listening, either in person, over the phone, or through video conferencing.

- **Nonverbal Communication**: Includes body language, facial expressions, gestures, and tone of voice, which often convey more than words alone.

- **Written Communication**: Encompasses emails, letters, reports, memos, and documentation, requiring careful consideration of language, tone, and clarity.

- **Visual Communication**: Utilizes visuals such as charts, graphs, diagrams, and presentations to convey information effectively.

4. Documentation:

- **Definition**: Documentation refers to the process of recording and preserving information in written, electronic, or visual formats.

- **Purpose**: Documentation serves various purposes, including record-keeping, information dissemination, legal compliance, and knowledge preservation.

- **Types of Documentation**: Examples include project plans, meeting minutes, technical specifications, policies and procedures, user manuals, and academic research papers.

- **Best Practices**: Clear, organized, and accurate documentation is crucial for ensuring accessibility, traceability, and accountability.

- **Tools**: Various tools and software, such as document management systems, wikis, and collaboration platforms, facilitate efficient documentation processes.

5. Importance of Documentation:

- **Legal Compliance**: Proper documentation ensures compliance with laws, regulations, and industry standards, reducing the risk of legal disputes or penalties.

- **Knowledge Management**: Documentation preserves institutional knowledge, allowing organizations to retain valuable information and expertise even as personnel change.

- **Decision-Making**: Well-documented information provides a basis for informed decision-making, strategic planning, and performance evaluation.

- **Communication Aid**: Documentation serves as a reference point for communication, enabling stakeholders to access relevant information as needed.

- **Risk Mitigation**: Comprehensive documentation helps identify and mitigate risks, errors, and discrepancies, promoting transparency and accountability.

6. Principles of Effective Documentation:

- **Accuracy**: Documentation should be factually correct and free from errors or misinformation.

- **Clarity**: Information should be presented clearly and logically, using language and terminology appropriate for the intended audience.

- **Consistency**: Maintaining consistency in formatting, style, and terminology enhances readability and usability.

- **Accessibility**: Documentation should be easily accessible to authorized users, whether in physical or digital formats, and searchable for quick reference.

- **Revision Control**: Implementing version control mechanisms ensures that documentation remains up-to-date and reflects the latest information.

Conclusion:

Communication and documentation are indispensable components of effective interaction and organizational management. By adhering to principles of clarity, accuracy, and accessibility, individuals and organizations can foster better understanding, collaboration, and success across various domains. Embracing best practices in communication and documentation empowers individuals and teams to achieve their goals, navigate challenges, and drive positive outcomes in today's interconnected world.

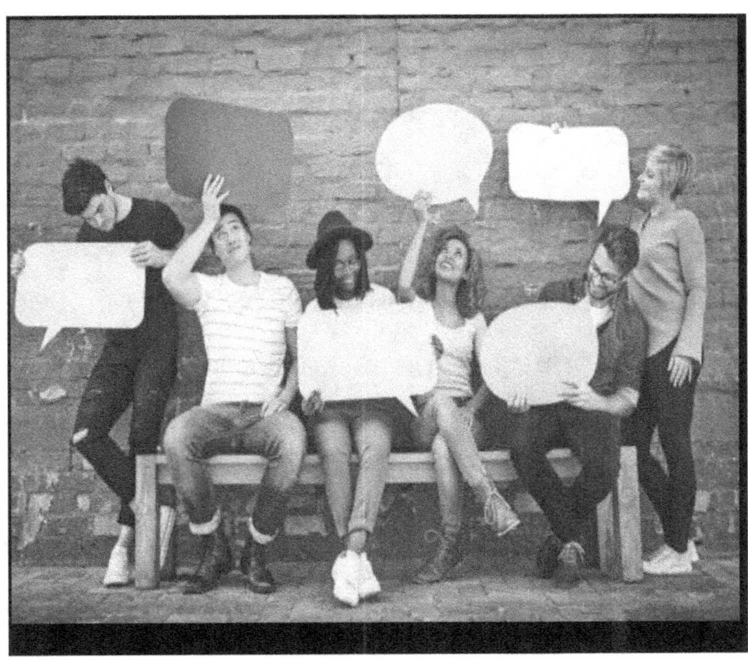

Communicating with Healthcare Providers

Introduction:

Effective communication with healthcare providers is essential for ensuring optimal healthcare outcomes. Whether you're visiting a doctor for a routine check-up, managing a chronic condition, or seeking treatment for an acute illness, clear and open communication is key to receiving the best possible care. In this guide, we'll explore various aspects of communicating with healthcare providers, including preparation for appointments, active listening techniques, asking questions, and advocating for your healthcare needs.

1. Preparation for Appointments:

- Make a list of your symptoms, concerns, and any questions you have before the appointment.

- Bring a list of medications you're currently taking, including over-the-counter drugs and supplements.

- Bring any relevant medical records, test results, or imaging reports.

- Arrive on time for your appointment to ensure you have enough time to discuss your concerns with your healthcare provider.

2. Active Listening Techniques:

- Listen attentively to your healthcare provider without interrupting.

- Take notes during the appointment to help you remember important information.

- Ask for clarification if you don't understand something your healthcare provider says.

- Summarize what you've understood to ensure you and your provider are on the same page.

3. Asking Questions:

- Don't be afraid to ask questions about your condition, treatment options, or any concerns you have.

- Use open-ended questions to encourage your healthcare provider to provide detailed responses.

- Write down any questions that arise during the appointment to ensure you don't forget to ask them.

- If you're unsure about a recommended treatment or medication, ask about potential side effects, alternatives, and the rationale behind the recommendation.

4. Advocating for Your Healthcare Needs:

- Be an active participant in your healthcare by expressing your preferences, concerns, and goals.

- If you feel uncomfortable with a proposed treatment plan, voice your concerns and discuss alternative options.

- If you're experiencing symptoms that aren't improving or worsening, don't hesitate to follow up with your healthcare provider.

- Seek a second opinion if you're uncertain about a diagnosis or treatment plan.

5. Communicating Effectively in Challenging Situations:

- If you're feeling overwhelmed or anxious, communicate this to your healthcare provider so they can provide support and reassurance.

- If you encounter communication barriers due to language or cultural differences, ask for interpretation services or cultural liaisons to facilitate communication.

- If you're facing financial constraints that impact your ability to adhere to a treatment plan, discuss this with your healthcare provider to explore alternative options.

Conclusion:

Effective communication with healthcare providers is vital for receiving high-quality care and achieving positive health outcomes. By preparing for appointments, actively listening, asking questions, advocating for your healthcare needs, and navigating challenging situations, you can ensure that your voice is heard and your concerns are addressed. Remember that your healthcare provider is there to help you, and open communication is the cornerstone of a successful patient-provider relationship.

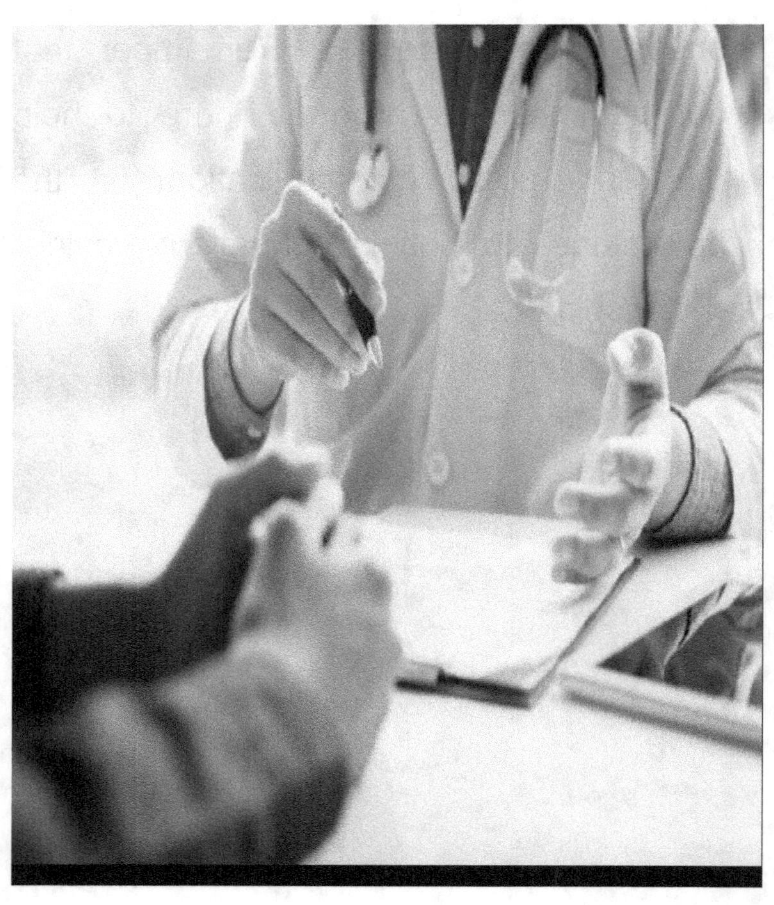

Documenting Symptoms and Progress

Introduction:

Documenting symptoms and progress is an essential aspect of managing health conditions, tracking recovery, and ensuring effective communication between patients and healthcare providers. Whether you're managing a chronic illness, recovering from an injury, or undergoing treatment for a medical condition, keeping detailed records can provide valuable insights into your health journey. This comprehensive guide explores the importance of documenting symptoms and progress, offers tips on how to do it effectively, and outlines what information to include.

Why Document Symptoms and Progress?

1. Facilitates Communication: Detailed records enable clear communication between patients and healthcare providers. When you can accurately describe your symptoms and progress, healthcare professionals can make more informed decisions about your care.

2. Tracks Changes Over Time: Documenting symptoms and progress allows you to track changes in your health over time. This longitudinal view can help identify patterns, triggers, and fluctuations in symptoms, providing valuable information for treatment adjustments.

3. Empowers Self-Advocacy: By documenting your experiences, you become an active participant in your healthcare journey. You can advocate for yourself more effectively, ask informed questions, and collaborate with healthcare providers to achieve the best possible outcomes.

4. Supports Treatment Planning: Healthcare providers rely on accurate information to develop effective treatment plans. Documenting symptoms and progress provides valuable data that can guide treatment decisions, medication adjustments, and lifestyle recommendations.

How to Document Symptoms and Progress:

1. Choose a Method: Find a documentation method that works for you. This could be a notebook, a health journal app, a spreadsheet, or even voice recordings. Choose a format that you're comfortable with and that you'll consistently use.

2. Be Consistent: Establish a routine for documenting symptoms and progress. Whether it's daily, weekly, or as needed, consistency is key to capturing accurate information and identifying trends over time.

3. Use Clear Language: Describe symptoms and experiences using clear, specific language. Include details such as severity, duration, frequency, and any factors that may influence symptoms (e.g., time of day, activities, triggers).

4. Include Relevant Information: In addition to symptoms, document other relevant information such as medication changes, treatments received, lifestyle factors (e.g., diet, exercise), and notable events (e.g., stressors, changes in routine).

5. Track Progress: Don't just focus on symptoms; also track progress and improvements. Note any positive changes, symptom relief strategies that work, and milestones reached in your health journey.

What to Include:

1. Date and Time: Record the date and time of each entry to track when symptoms occur and how they change over time.

2. Symptom Description: Describe each symptom in detail, including its nature, intensity, duration, and any associated factors or triggers.

3. Medications and Treatments: Document any medications taken, dosage changes, or treatments received, including their effectiveness and any side effects experienced.

4. Lifestyle Factors: Note relevant lifestyle factors such as diet, exercise, sleep patterns, stress levels, and any changes that may impact your symptoms.

5. Emotional and Mental Health: Consider documenting your emotional and mental health alongside physical symptoms. This can provide a more comprehensive view of your overall well-being.

6. Questions and Concerns: Use your documentation to jot down questions, concerns, or topics you want to discuss with your healthcare provider during appointments.

Conclusion:

Documenting symptoms and progress is a valuable tool for managing health conditions, tracking recovery, and enhancing communication with healthcare providers. By establishing a consistent documentation routine, using clear language, and including relevant information, you can gain insights into your health journey, advocate for yourself more effectively, and collaborate with healthcare providers to achieve optimal outcomes. Whether you prefer pen and paper or digital tools, find a method that works for you and commit to documenting your experiences. It's an investment in your health and well-being.

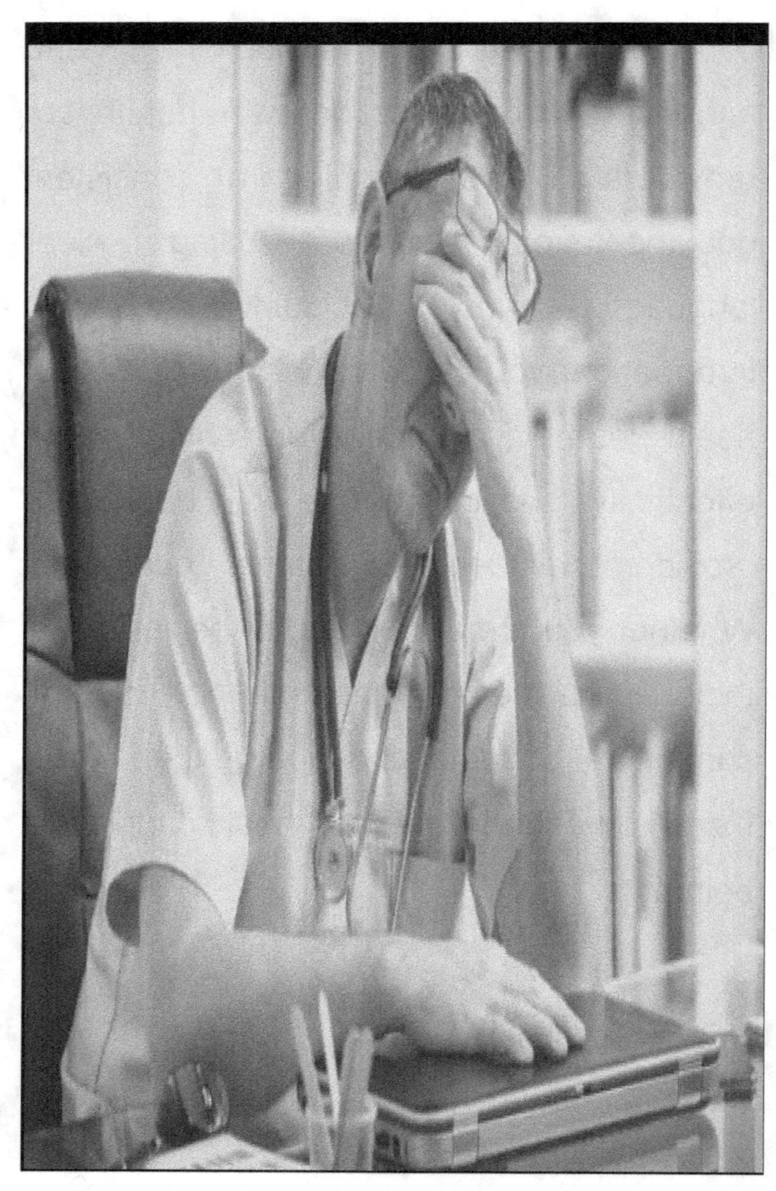

www.ingramcontent.com/pod-product-compliance
Lightning Source LLC
Chambersburg PA
CBHW071223260726
48653CB00042B/1810